THE JOURNEY

PRINCIPLES OF TOTAL LIFE TRANSFORMATION

THE JOURNEY

PRINCIPLES OF TOTAL LIFE TRANSFORMATION

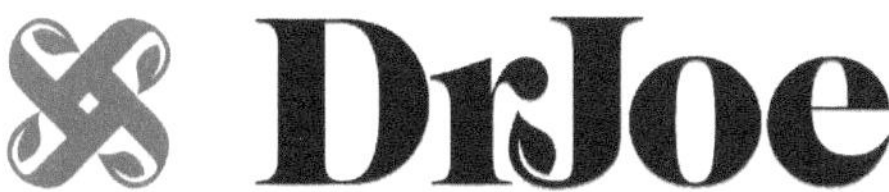

TABLE OF CONTENTS

Part 1: The Opportunity.........................7

Introduction...................................9

Chapter 1: Obstacles of the Mind and Body...........11

Chapter 2: Obstacles of the Spirit.................29

Part 2: My Journey............................39

Chapter 3: How It All Started 41

Chapter 4: Jumping into the Journey 53

Chapter 5: What I Learned......................59

Part 3: It's Your Turn.........................67

Chapter 6: The 10 Laws of Personal Transformation......69

Chapter 7: Always Live in Reality.................83

Conclusion...................................93

PART 1
THE OPPORTUNITY

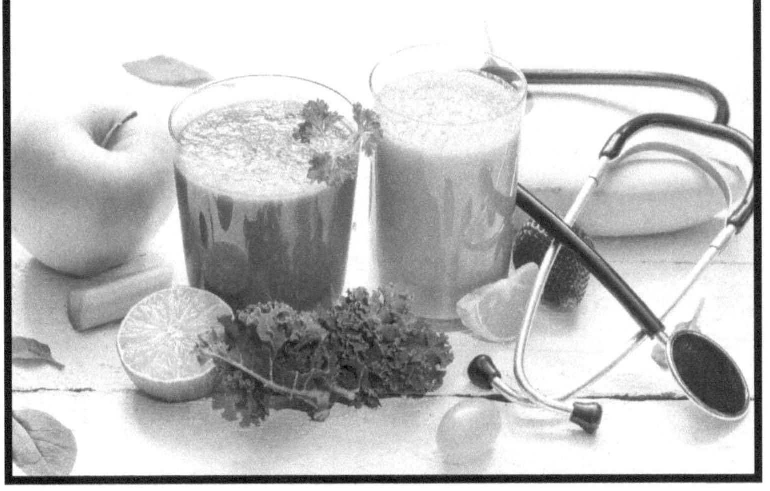

INTRODUCTION

All men and women are created equal; however, all men and women are not equal in their ability to maximize their life. Why is it that some succeed while others fail? Why is success such a rarity, while failure seems abundant? Why do people spend their lives looking for "the way," but rarely seem to find it?

The answers to these questions are found deep within the soul of every man and woman. We each must take a journey inside of ourselves in order to unlock the mysteries of life, and find the answers for which we're searching.

God made us all the same; however, the journey we take to become our best includes a different path for each of us. When we understand that what we're really looking for is found deep within, we find direction and opportunity to become the very best version of ourselves!

Fear of Change

Homeostasis is "the ability to maintain a relatively stable internal state that persists despite changes in the world outside. All living organisms, from plants to puppies to people, must regulate their internal environment to process energy and ultimately survive." [1] Although this is a biological term, the concept of homeostasis is something for which all human beings have a natural proclivity. We have a desire to maintain consistency in all areas of our existence, whether they be

---

[1] Lanese, Nicoletta. "What is Homeostasis?" Livescience.com. https://www. livescience.com/65938-homeostasis.html (accessed December 24, 2019).

biological, social, or physical. This part of us makes change difficult.

Losing weight, breaking habits, changing how we think, or even being consistent with a new habit are simple concepts that are surprisingly hard to implement. Change is hard for us because, at our core, we desire the comfort of consistency more than the joy of transformation. It's only when we understand this that sustainable and consistent transformation can begin to take place.

Obstacles of Transformation

You have an opportunity not only to change who you are, but to understand the major obstacles that impede personal transformation. The Journey is a spiritual process that takes us deep within, in order to find personal change. Many times, people change without truly understanding the obstacles that make this process so challenging; however, you have the opportunity here to understand what you're doing. The knowledge you gain will help you not only on your personal journey, but in any goal or desire you have in your life. There are three main obstacles to transformation of any kind. In the next couple of chapters, we're going to examine each one in detail.

Chapter 1

OBSTACLES OF THE MIND AND BODY

The first obstacles to transformation that we're going to examine are those that occur in our minds. All emotions, reactions, and experiences have their genesis within the mind. What you are living—your reality—is nothing more than an interpretation. This means that individuals can have the same circumstances and wildly different experiences. The mind is a powerful computer that creates reality. What we think is "real" is nothing more than a projection of our own mental state. When you understand the power of the mind, you will understand the importance of changing how you think.

The mind creating reality is a philosophy that intersects with both religious and non-religious beliefs. The Bible says, "For as he thinks in his heart, so is he."[2] There have been several writings unrelated to any major religion that share similar sentiments. Understanding the power of the mind, what it does, and how it creates our reality is important when journeying down the road of transformation. There are important functions of the mind that we must know, understand, and use for our benefit whenever transformation is our goal. The important functions of the mind include its ability to react to and interpret things.

---

[2] New King James Version. Proverbs 23:7

Interpretation

What we deem as reality is nothing more than how the mind interprets what we see or experience. Based on our past, what we know and how we perceive things will determine how we interpret them. For example, if two children are raised in the same household, and the parents of those children decide to divorce, the actions could impact both children differently. One child may grow up so concerned about not reliving divorce that he does all he can to ensure that his marriage never ends in divorce; however, the other child may grow up fearing divorce because of the pain she experienced. This fear may cause the second child to avoid marriage in order to avoid the pain of divorce.

Within this example, there is one action—divorce; however, the two children have different interpretations. Both realities had different results—how the children thought, reacted, and responded. Their entire lives were affected based upon how they interpreted one event.

Reality is not about what is, but rather how the mind interprets it. Reality is created within the mind by way of interpretation; it's something that occurs subconsciously. When we become aware of the power of the mind, we find the ability to make any situation what we desire it to be by how we interpret what is happening.

For example, if I am a person who is without something in my life (e.g., a father, friends, the means to get the things I want, etc.), I can use those things as deliberate motivating factors to seek and become whatever I desire to be. Instead of interpreting myself as a victim, I can use the power of my mind to become motivated to improve my life. A man raised without his father can either blame his struggles in life on not having a father (victim mentality), or he can make a decision to be the very best father he can be for his own child. He can intentionally use not having a father as motivation to become a good father.

Within various sports leagues (NFL, NBA, MLB, NHL), the season always ends with a clash between the two top teams to see who is the best. The final game comes after multiple rounds of eliminations, and usually pits the "favorite" team against the "underdog" team. Great teams of the past have been able to draw strength from being in the position of the underdog. Being thought of as the team that will lose isn't admirable; however, the mind can make its own reality by intentionally interpreting the status of "underdog" as a positive! It can draw inspiration, motivation, and energy from being underestimated in order to overcome a major obstacle (the opposing team). Likewise, we can do the same in any situation, at any time we desire. The key is being aware of what you think, and intentionally using the power of interpretation to create whatever reality you choose, regardless of the situation or circumstance.

There are steps that need to be taken in order to implement this. When you understand these steps, it will make the practice more usable and effective. First, before you can interpret a situation from the vantage point that is most advantageous to you spiritually, mentally, and emotionally, you must understand the limitless nature of emotions. As your feelings ebb and flow, you must interact with them accordingly.

Emotional Awareness

When you have a feeling, no matter how good or bad it is, you must first understand what it is. Emotions and feelings are like visitors to a house—they come and go. Some stay longer than others; however, at some point, each one will leave. When you understand this, you will understand that emotions have no permanence within our mind.

This is beneficial in the case of bad emotions because when you experience fear, angst, or confusion, you can know that these feelings are psychological responses to what you perceive. When you are aware of your feelings and redirect your focus, what you feel will change. This fact is also beneficial in the case of good emotions because their coming and going reminds us that, rather than being merely a result of circumstances, joy and happiness are states within which we choose to exist.

When you have a feeling, understand it for what it is. We should never treat emotions as something of permanence, especially when their causes are external events or circumstances. The danger of not understanding the nature of emotions comes when we make decisions or take actions solely based on how we feel. For example, when anger enters your heart and you act as a result of it, most of the time you will regret what you do. On the other hand, the emotion that has been observed and acknowledged for what it is empowers us to act wisely, because we know it will eventually dissipate and leave. We can control the effects that our emotions have on us by simply being aware of them as they visit our heart and mind.

Refocus

When we have become aware of our emotions, the next step is to refocus our attention. This is critical. When a negative emotion comes and we are aware of it, we must refocus our mind. The place of our focus should be in the direction that's desirable—not where we are, but where we desire to be. For example, if I receive a call that my business venture is failing, my mind can intentionally focus on finding solutions instead of dwelling on the problem. When we dwell within negativity, nothing good ever comes of it; however, when our thoughts are refocused onto something that we can control, the outcome is much more productive.

Like a trained fighter who takes punches while remaining focused on his strategy, we should be aware of our emotions without breaking focus on what we need to accomplish. Life will throw many punches; however, when they come, we must understand our ability to choose how we react. We have more power than we often understand.

What is the importance of refocusing? The quality of what we do is directly connected to our mental and emotional state. Most times, the better your state of being, the better you are able to work—and the higher quality work you are able to produce. Most people allow their state to be shifted based on temporary emotions and circumstances; however, we must understand, even in the midst of undesirable circumstances, that we can refocus and redirect our thoughts onto the solution.

Recenter

As a plane flies high above the ground, it encounters a multitude of challenges and obstacles. When turbulence comes, the plane's systems notify the pilot. At this moment, the pilot realizes she has a choice: should I remain at this altitude or move from where I am? This is the moment she becomes aware. Once this occurs, the pilot will redirect the plane to a higher or lower altitude. Her desire isn't to remain where she is, but to find another place where the air is not rough—she refocuses herself and her plane. The pilot continues to climb or descend until the rough air is left behind. Then she levels the plane and remains at that altitude until something else occurs. This is called recentering.

Air travel is a continual, circular process of awareness, refocusing, and recentering. This happens over and over again throughout daily air travel. This process also occurs with us. Once we are aware of our emotions and we have refocused our thoughts, our life will recenter, allowing us to function in an undisturbed state of being. The person who masters this process of not allowing temporary emotional states to become permanent states of being is the person who can master the act of living! Just as with anything else, the more this is done, the easier it becomes.

Reactions of the Mind

If you reflect upon the issues and struggles you've experienced in your past, chances are that 99% of them are the result of how you responded to a certain person, action, or circumstance. Many times, these responses are subconscious. As a child, I remember that whenever I was on a plane, I had an overwhelming sense of fear and anxiety. Likewise, whenever

I found myself at high elevations—on the sides of mountains or even traveling up or down an elevator—my fear felt overwhelming. In most instances, I didn't know why I felt as I did. I blamed it on having a fear of heights. Within my mind, I was okay with that classification. I felt that I could live my life around my fears by simply avoiding heights.

This is typical within our society. When we have issues or problems, we are quick to diagnose them or have someone diagnosis us. Most of the time, however, the process of diagnosis is nothing more than taking those with certain symptoms and placing them into a group with others who possess the same symptoms. This could be the diagnosis process for depression, fear, obesity, or a litany of other ailments. From the time of diagnosis, the patient is taught how to cope with their issue through medication or perhaps treatment. Seldom are we aware of the power of the mind, and how it creates problems that we simply accept and hold onto for years—sometimes, even a lifetime.

But what if I were able to understand the issues behind my apparent fear of heights? What if I were able to see that my fears were merely born from fabrications of my mind, reinforced by my acceptance of being a person who is afraid of heights? All the fears that you have at this moment were created in your mind. They were made by your mind—in many instances, subconsciously, through repetition. We train ourselves to be slaves of the mind, which creates these realities we feel we must accept.

Joseph Murphy puts it this way: "Once the subconscious mind accepts an idea, it begins to execute it. It is an astonishing and subtle truth that the law of the subconscious mind works for good and bad ideas alike. This law, when applied in a negative way, is the cause of failure, frustration, and unhappiness. When your habitual thinking is harmonious and constructive, however, you experience perfect health, success, and prosperity."[3]

The biggest truth surrounding the mind's power is that it creates reality unknowingly, or subconsciously. This can be dangerous as well as inefficient—dangerous because there are a multitude of negative experiences that we could have avoided by being aware of our mind's power; inefficient because, if we are unaware of what the mind is able to accomplish, we will not use its power to maximize our abilities. Instead, we will remain prisoners of the mind's tricks and reactions to things, people, and circumstances.

For years I had a car; however, I never took time to read the owner's manual. There was a button in the center console that had an icon of a car with small lines alongside the rear tires. I never knew what it was supposed to indicate. One day, I pressed the button; to my surprise, the transmission became sharper, and the exhaust note became louder. The car was a completely different car than before—it had more abilities and powers than I'd realized! When I researched the button, I learned that it activated a sport mode. Once I learned what it did and how to use it, I had a different experience with my car. Likewise, when we understand the power of the mind, we move into a place in which we're able to have a different experience in life; we are able to control situations that once controlled us; we are able to mitigate issues that once derailed our progress and direction.

---

[3] Murphy, Joseph "The Power of your Subconscious Mind." Pg. 16-17. Prentice Hall Press. 2008.

The part of the mind that creates issues, the subconscious mind, is a real part of us; it's valuable, but it can also create problems. It's the source of the feelings and mood swings we can see, even when we don't understand what they mean or why we're experiencing them. But the mind reacts in the way *we train it* to react. Our reactions are actually based upon a three-stage process: the planting of a seed, the growth of the roots, and the manifestation of the fruit.

The Seed

Earlier, I shared with you about my fear of heights. All of my life, I accepted the fact that I was afraid of heights; however, I never understood that my fear was a creation of my mind. I subconsciously trained myself to react to heights as I did. My fear began with the planting of a seed. All states of being for that matter—phobias, fears, anxiety, trust issues, addictions—start with a seed planted deep within our subconscious mind.

As a child, I remembered traveling with my mother. Whenever we found ourselves on planes, she would always respond in fear when the plane experienced any level of turbulence. The look of terror on her face bothered me to the depths of my soul. Every time we flew, my mother was in a constant state of fear from takeoff to landing. There was never a time when she wasn't afraid. I'm not blaming my mother for her subconscious state of fear; but it was at that time when my own seed of fear was planted into my subconscious mind. I was trained from a young age by someone I love dearly to fear heights! This is a common occurrence in life. People project their fears onto us, most of the time without realizing what they are doing. It's likely that if you have a fear of death, failure, divorce, relationships, loneliness, and so on, that these states of being are nothing more than seeds that were once planted into your mind.

Take time to think about, and maybe even write down, the issues you perceive in and around your life. Perhaps you have ways of viewing certain people or situations that you know aren't normal. If you take time to analyze these issues, you can usually trace them back to the moment the seed was planted into your subconscious mind.

Children who are abused oftentimes grow up to become abusive adults, or adults who never reach a certain level of maturity. Trauma and stress have effects on brain development and the way we process information. I was taught to be afraid of heights—to react in a certain way and at a certain time. My mother's response to heights was a seed planted early on in my childhood.

The point is this: the mind is a powerful tool that we often don't foster with intention. Most people allow what others do to set the trajectory of how they respond. It seems normal to panic when we are jobless, or to cry when someone passes away. I'm not saying those responses are wrong; however, I'm saying that we subconsciously teach ourselves how to react and respond to certain situations.

Growth of the Roots

Once a seed is planted, it establishes roots. Whatever grows in the future will be located at the place where the seed was planted. The older I became, the more I reinforced my fear of heights by continually repeating the same things I'd seen in my mother's behavior. I would become afraid whenever I was on a plane taking off; whenever we encountered turbulence; whenever we descended to land. The more I flew, and the more I reenacted this emotion, the more I found myself doing the same things over and over again. When I would go onto elevators, escalators, or anything that was elevated, I would experience the same fears. My issues weren't isolated to the plane; instead, they expanded to other places and situations. The seed that had been planted into my mind was establishing roots in my subconscious. I was slowly becoming something I did not understand.

This is how the mind becomes our biggest hindrance in life. I created my own fear—my own phobia of height. As time progressed, the seed's grip on my mind led to an inability to control my mind. Now that I understand more about the power of my mind, I realize that my fears were projections which created my own reality.

Think about your life, and how many seeds have been planted into your subconscious mind. Perhaps you've had seeds of jealously, envy, wrong eating habits, abuse, anger, fear, or failure planted. There can also be many positive seeds. The key to the mind is not its different responses to good or bad seeds, but rather the truth that any planted seed will grow and establish roots. Flaws within our character, such as narcissism, addiction, eating disorders, and a variation of phobias are nothing more than seeds that have established roots. We become what we've allowed to grow. The reason many people aren't able to kick certain habits or change certain behaviors is that they attempt to change their physical environment without understanding the importance of identifying the seed—the roots—of the problem.

The Fruit

Before an apple becomes a fruit, it is a seed. Before the apple tree sprouts from beneath the ground where it was planted, it grows under the surface. Likewise, this happens within us. We possess many things that start as seeds within our minds: personalities, character traits, and so on. Long before we became who we are, these seeds were planted—in many instances, without our awareness. After a time, the seed grows and establishes roots. One day, we become who we are.

Many people believe that who we are is merely a combination of genes and random occurrences. We accept our identities as something out of our control—something we're unable to change. We buy into the mantra that "This is just who I am." This does two things. First of all, it refuses personal responsibility for what we have become. Secondly, it creates complacency, because "who I am" cannot be changed. People then become the very things they unknowingly create for themselves in their perceived reality.

As we grow, our objective should be to not allow negative seeds to manifest, and to be more mindful about planting positive seeds that will reap the harvest we truly desire.

Obstacles of the Body

If you watch any TV, online stream, or social media site, you'll see hundreds of people either struggling with weight issues or selling products to help people with weight issues. Weight, along with the desire for better health, is something that transcends race, religion, and location. It is an issue that has become more problematic today than ever before.

The obstacles of the body primarily result not from physical problems, but rather our lack of understanding as to who we are, as well as the structure of society. When we understand how modern society is not conducive to the health of the human body, we can begin to remove those obstacles and manifest the change we desire. Let's take a look at just a few of the obstacles to bodily health in our society today.

The largest obstacle to physical health, especially in Western cultures, is our relationship with food. In the West, food is used to meet needs that it was not designed to meet. It's used to celebrate—when someone is married, when a baby is born, we eat. It's used to mourn—when someone passes away, we eat. Customs and food go hand and hand. This mindset gives food purposes besides its original divine purpose.

What is that divine purpose? The purpose of food is to sustain life—it's not something that should aid in a celebration or cultural ritual. When we understand our cultural patterns of using food for celebratory means instead of what it was designed for, we can see how our culture has created obstacles that impede ideal weight and health.

The Size of Meals

We eat entirely too much! Food is always prepared and ready for consumption. It can be found in the local grocery store, in the pantry of every home, and in break rooms in corporate offices and schools everywhere. We are constantly eating; and when we aren't eating, we're thinking about what we will eat next.

Our cultural mindset towards food causes us to have a bad relationship with something that was designed to give us optimal health and wellbeing. When we go to restaurants, we desire large servings. A new study, published in *The Journal of the American Academy of Nutrition and Dietetics*, looked at meals served at 123 restaurants in three cities across America. As it turns out, single-meal servings—*excluding* beverages, appetizers, and desserts—exceeded recommended calorie requirements in most cases. In fact, single meals sometimes exceeded the caloric requirements for an entire day![4]

Overeating has become an American way of living. This is a major obstacle, because the basic function of food is to provide energy. The energy that we eat is the power that moves all things down to our very cells. When we overeat, the body is taxed and unable to process what we have given it. When you fill up your car with too much gas, the fuel overflows. For humans, this overflow manifests through the process of gaining weight. Higher levels of obesity in the West are largely due to us overeating.

Americans have a hard time with diets because the amount of food needed for healthy lifestyles is vastly lower than "normal" portions. For this reason, many people feel extreme hunger when on a diet, when in actuality, the smaller portions are in alignment with what the body was designed to consume.

Observing a baby and his or her frequency of eating gives insight to the proper portions for human consumption. When baby is born, it will desire to nurse every 2-3 hours. The mother produces just enough milk to sustain the child for this period of time. As the child rests, the mother's milk supply replenishes. In another 2-3 hours, the baby will repeat the process. The baby is never given an overabundance of milk—just what it needs to promote growth and development. I'm not suggesting we should eat like babies, but I do think reassessing portions is essential for us in order to remove the obstacles that make us culturally predisposed to obesity.

---

[4] Swerdoff, Alex. "92 Percent of America's Restaurants Serve Oversized Portions" www.vice.com. https://www.vice.com/en_us/article/78dkzq/92-percent-of-americas-restaurants-serve-oversized-portions. Accessed Jan. 3, 2020.

Frequency of Eating

Secondly, we eat too often! American culture is obsessed with the concept of snacking. A typical American way of eating is to start with breakfast, followed by a snack. This is followed by lunch, and then another a snack—same thing for dinner. The body is constantly in a state of being fed. There is never a period of fasting until nighttime, when we are asleep. When large meals are coupled with a high frequency of eating, it creates a soup that will lead to sickness and obesity. When the body is constantly being fed, it means energy is constantly being used to break down food.

Think of it like this. If you use your entire income up on buying things, what will you do when an appliance needs to be fixed, or a roof needs to be replaced? You won't have funds to address these problems when they arise. Energy in the body works the same way. There's only so much energy we have; and when we are constantly in a state of being overfed, the body is using an abundance of energy on digesting food. The energy you need to recover, heal, and recuperate is often used up on digestion, resulting in sluggishness, aches, and pains through-out the body. Sometimes, the best healing for the body comes when we abstain from food. Fasting is not a popular subject within a culture constantly eating, but it's an important one nonetheless.

Made to Move

Human beings were made to run, jump, climb, and swim. The bodies we possess are designed to move. This is an obstacle for us, because our society lives sedentary lives which lead to disease and cardiovascular issues—problems that could be prevented with small adjustments! From sitting in front of computers for eight hours a day to constantly looping around parking lots just to find that space close to the front door, we're doing all we can to avoid moving, and it's literally killing us.

Living a sedentary life means we don't get the exercise we need to optimize our lives. When you live an active life, it removes obstacles that keep us from a healthy, sustainable life. Let's clarify something though: an active lifestyle doesn't necessarily mean going to the gym 2-3 times per week. It simply means physically exerting yourself every day! People's assumptions about what constitutes being active cause them to conclude that it's too much effort. However, these assumptions are formed by a sedentary society! When we make the effort to live an active lifestyle, the following benefits begin to show up in our lives.

Improved Cardiovascular Health

When you live a sedentary life, the blood vessels, capillaries, and veins responsible for moving blood around the body become constricted. These pathways were made to contract and expand. When expansion and contraction are frequent—in an active lifestyle—the functionality of the circulatory system improves. With physical exertion, the heart is trained to become more efficient. The heartbeat of a trained athlete is actually slower than the heartbeat of someone who is sedentary. This conditioning process has many health benefits that we do not experience as a society due to our sedentary lifestyles.

Improved Mood

Depression, anxiety, and other forms of mental illness are common ailments in American society. The number of people who suffer from these conditions increases each year. A sedentary lifestyle doesn't help improve mental health; in fact, in many ways, it makes it worse. Living an active lifestyle not only gives us the physical health benefits we desire, but it also has a great impact on our mental health and wellness in the following ways:

- Exercise helps depression because it causes the body to release serotonin, a chemical that regulates mood
- Exercise helps to flush out chemicals that can contribute to depression
- Exercise helps to establish our sleep schedule
- Exercise helps to alleviate stress[5]

Many people who struggle with depression and anxiety can instantly improve their mental state by incorporating daily exercise into their lifestyle. Exercise can eliminate the need for many prescription drugs used to balance out the chemicals in the brain. Movement is essential to human health, because we're designed to move daily.

Lower Rates of Obesity

Obesity numbers continue to rise year after year. There are many preventable diseases connected to high levels of obesity, such as heart disease, diabetes, and even cancer. Most people who struggle with obesity haven't committed themselves to daily, vigorous exercise. When we make a commitment to move regularly, we can eliminate obesity by reversing the sedentary nature of the society in which we live.

According to the Centers for Disease Control and Prevention, "More than 100 million U.S. adults are now living with

---

[5] No author's name was given "Exercise and Mood" www.betterhealth.vic.gov.au https://www.betterhealth.vic.gov.au/health/HealthyLiving/exercise-and-moodaccessed Jan. 4, 2020.

diabetes or pre-diabetes."[6] This means that 1 in 3 people in the United States are suffering from a disease that, in most instances, can be fully controlled by lifestyle. Why is this percentage so high? Because of the things we've just mentioned: the size of our meals, the frequency of those meals, and our overall sedentary lifestyle. By removing these obstacles of the body, we can bring health to individuals and our society as a whole.

---

[6] More than 100 million Americans have diabetes or pre-diabetes. www.cdc. gov. https://www.cdc.gov/media/releases/2017/p0718-diabetes-report.html.

Chapter 2

OBSTACLES OF THE SPIRIT

The spirit is arguably the most difficult aspect of health for us to address. Many people agree that we possess a spirit; however, we don't always understand what it does, or even how it works. When you turn on a computer, you press a button and simply wait for it to power on. You email, surf the web, video message various people, and so on; however, what do you do when it breaks? It's hard to know what's wrong with it, or what needs fixing.

The spirit is the most neglected part of man's being. Why? Because it's the complete antithesis of the way our society is living. Life in our culture is a physical experience first; this is why we often forget about our spiritual essence. When a person is looking to change or address an issue (e.g. addiction, obesity, depression, etc.), the normal methods suggested by society don't include caring for the spirit at all. For example, if a person struggles to lose weight and tries a variety of diets without success, they'll often conclude that nothing works for them. But why is it that nothing ever worked? Many times, it's because the issues aren't with the physical body, but rather in the spiritual essence of the person. Obstacles of the spirit manifest in a few primary ways; let's take a look at them together.

Lack of Understanding the Spirit

One day while driving down the highway, I set my cruise control to 55 miles per hour. Ten miles down the road, a police officer pulled me over. When he pulled me over, he told me, "Sir, you've been speeding." I was surprised, and thought there must be a mistake. I told him that my cruise control was set to 55 miles per hour. The police officer looked at me and said, "Sir, for the past five miles, the speed limit is 40 miles per hour." I was shocked, and found myself in trouble because I was unaware of the speed limit.

When we are unaware of our spiritual essence—what it is and how it works—we can find ourselves entrenched in issues without knowing why we are there or how to get out. These can be struggles such as addiction, fear, depression, anxiety… the list goes on. All these things are impacted by spiritual elements of life. How does the spirit impact physical reality? This question needs to be answered in order to bring about an understanding of why the spirit cannot be neglected when we're looking to transform.

When you watch a movie at a theatre, you give your attention to the screen. All of the action, drama, and suspense is there, after all. However, the actual image you see is a projection—it's coming from a different place. In actuality, the image is coming from behind you, not in front of you. The projector is to the movie what the spirit is to our lives. Every issue and problem you have ever grappled with starts within your spiritual essence, and the state of your spirit is projected onto everything you do.

My fear of heights was a seed that affected my thoughts and actions; it caused me to project a reality that was from deep within—from a spiritual place. Once we understand that our spirit is where problems begin, we can take a new approach to transformation and change. There are many people who struggle with losing weight, no matter what they try. Sometimes their problems are made worse when they see others succeed with certain programs or diets, and they aren't able to follow suit. You cannot support a person like this by giving them another diet. Why? Because the *diet* only caters to the physical part of that person.

Most times in my experience, when people are unable to lose weight, the issue is spiritual. These individuals have learned (subconsciously) to eat when they reach a certain emotional state. Food is a tool to help them cope with life's situations. When you understand the spiritual manifestation of this, you'll learn how to address the issue not physically, but spiritually. When the body is addressed and the spirit is neglected, temporary results ensue. A person will lose weight and feel good about themselves for a short period of time if they try hard enough; however, at a certain point, the person slowly returns to who they've always been. Habits will return, and the result they initially received will be lost—they'll be back at square one.

However, when the spirit of a person is addressed in the transformative process, it becomes a holistic process, because the root cause is discovered. This process occurs in three steps.

Step 1: Identify the Issue

The first step of transformation is identifying the emotion connected to the desire. In other words, if a person is an emotional eater, they must identify what emotion causes them to want to eat. Sometimes, this emotion can be a negative one (stress, fear, anxiety, etc.). Other times, the emotion can be a positive one (celebration, being in love, happiness, etc.). Whether the emotion is good or bad isn't important during this step. The important thing is to identify what it is, so that you can be aware of the underlying cause.

When the issue is identified, the person has a target to aim for in their desire to change. They are aware of the root and are able to focus their thoughts and actions on changing it.

Step 2: Isolate and Address the Emotion

Once the emotion is identified, it must be addressed, processed, and properly put in perspective. Emotional eaters eat because they are attempting to deal with their emotions by doing something that makes them feel better. When the emotion is identified, they can address it for what it is instead of responding to it subconsciously.

If you eat when you're stressed, the goal is to simply become aware of the times when you feel stressed. Getting in the habit of identifying stress allows you to become aware of it the moment it arises. If your emotion is properly tracked, you'll start to notice patterns throughout the course of a day or week. This becomes a powerful weapon—now you're able to identify the times of day when you're typically (subconsciously) moved to eat.

Step 3: Address and Redirect

Once someone has identified and isolated the issue, they're able to intentionally redirect their focus to something besides eating. They are now in a position of power. Most times, when the issue is identified, the desire to eat can be controlled. The person is able to redirect their thoughts, change their focus, and intentionally do something else that will address their feelings.

This approach can be used with any issue of the spirit. After all, eating isn't the only habit people have as a manifestation of a spiritual issue. The key is understanding that the root cause is an issue of the spirit that manifests in the body. When this is understood, issues can be addressed accordingly.

A Lack of Purging the Spirit

Most people are familiar with the concept of detoxing. This is a process whereby the body is cleansed of impurities. It can happen over the course of a day, a week, or any other specific amount of time. People who have detoxed attest that they feel better, lighter, and more full of energy. Most times, the term is used in a physical context.

Just like the body needs cleansing, the spirit does, also. We are exposed to things each and every day, by way of TV, work, home, relationships, and other sources. Seeds of anger, aggressiveness, and negativity can be planted on a daily basis. When we come away from these environments, many of us never take time to purge ourselves from the manifestation of these things.

When anything is inundated with waste or something it was not made to absorb, there is always some sort of buildup. When a buildup is not addressed and cleansed, malfunction will ultimately occur. When we look at our society, we can see evidence of people who need to clean themselves spiritually.

Steps to Cleanse One's Spirit

When a drain is clogged, the first thing we need do is stop the flow of water. Every day, we need to be in environments in which what we listen to and see is filtered. This will stop the buildup of things that create spiritual waste.

According to *The New York Post,* "A study by global tech protection and support company Asurion found that the average person struggles to go little more than 10 minutes without checking their phone. And of the 2,000 people surveyed, one in 10 check their phones on average once every four minutes." [7] This is a new phenomenon that is only worsening as time progresses. As people constantly check their phones and "connect" with friends and family via social media, they're inundated with fake lifestyles and constant opportunities to compare themselves with those they see. This creates feelings of failure, jealousy, envy, and an overall sense of unhappiness. On a daily basis, people need to remove themselves from these kinds of environments in order to purge any places that may create a toxic buildup of waste.

Once the things that have clogged the drain are filtered, it's time to clean the drain. When we avoid things that "clog us up" spiritually, it allows our spirit to be cleansed. How do we cleanse our spirit? By connecting ourselves to things that feed and nurture our spirit. Meditation, prayer, and journaling are just a few examples of these practices. When this is done consistently and with intention, people feel a reconnection with themselves—the things that blocked the spirit were the same items keeping the person from their true, authentic selves.

---

[7] "Americans check their phones 80 times a day." www.nypost.com https://nypost.com/2017/11/08/americans-check-their-phones-80-times-a-day-study/.

Once a drain is cleansed, there has to be a process of intentional maintenance to prevent future clogs and buildup. As spiritual beings, we need to detoxify ourselves spiritually on a consistent basis. As we mature, we understand that a clean spirit is an essential part of empowered living. The more we give attention to our spirit, the better our physical life will be.

The Spiritual Impact on the Body

A person's desire to change starts from within. Change is about controlling those things that affect us spiritually. Only then can we move forward with intention and live the kind of life we desire. Although the body and the spirit are separate entities, they do have places of intersection.

Think about a connection on a highway, where one major highway intersects with another. There is a point where they share a common space. Likewise, this occurs within each of us. Every day, in innumerable situations, your spirit and body intersect. When something makes you upset, you can feel your body heating up. When you hear bad news, you can feel a drop in your stomach. Your spirit and mind are intertwined and connected on a multitude of levels. This being the case, we must understand how the body impacts the spirit by way of diet and nutrition. When the body is fed foods that are heavy, greasy, oily, and void of nutrition, the spirit will suffer.

For this reason, diet and nutrition is a tool that must be used if you want to reach higher states of spiritual awareness. Throughout the Bible, we see the concept of how Christ fasted for days at a time, denying himself food and other things, all to gain spiritual insight or power. When you look at examples like this, and when you understand how the body and spirit are connected through nutrition, you can see how nutrition can be used as a tool.

If a person wants to transform themselves, they must start with changing their diet first! The diet must be full of clean foods that are full of nutrition, not processed, and eaten in the proper portion sizes. When a person is given these types of foods, it will empower them to see their way more clearly. Their mood and outlook will shift in a positive manner. They will lose weight and have a different understanding of themselves. Inflammation in the body will decrease, and the process of healing will create a spiritual power that carries over in ways that many do not even understand. When we understand how the body and spirit intersect by way of nutrition, it should cause us to view every form of "treatment" differently than we do. For alcoholics, drug addicts, people who are depressed, divorcees looking for change, and any person who has a problem they desire help with, the first step of true healing starts with changing the person's nutritional profile.

I've worked with people who suffer from all of these issues; although they have different problems, the root cause is the same: their spirit needs to be cleaned and detoxified. This cannot be done without knowledge of diet and nutrition, along with an awareness of the physical and spiritual intersections. When we understand both the body and the spirit, and how nutrition plays an essential role for both, we can begin to change our ways, and transformation can manifest.

Your Opportunity

I haven't been able to find anything I have shared with you elsewhere. The knowledge I've received is wisdom, awareness gained through experience. When I started ministry at the age of 21, I never saw myself doing what I am today. When I entered into the field of health and wellness, I never wanted to be the "healthy preacher." The more I did transformative work—using diet and nutrition as a tool and cornerstone in my approach—the more I felt as if my spiritual background as a pastor was in competition with it.

In time, I began to see how spirituality and health are perfect complements! You have the opportunity to understand this philosophy as well, and apply it to yourself. You can learn from what I had to discover on my own. In the next section of this book, I will share my story, and how I was transformed. See if you can find any similarities between my story and your own; for, although we all have different stories, we are all made up of the same essence. This means that our approach to living an empowered life will be similar, and not as different as we might think.

PART 2
MY JOURNEY

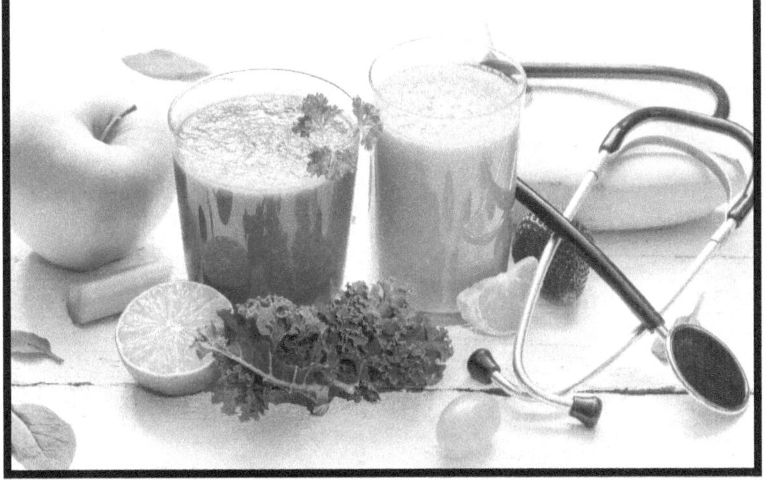

Chapter 3

HOW IT ALL STARTED

As a child, I was always actively involved in sports. Any sport that allowed me to compete and be part of a team intrigued me. My favorite was football—I loved it more than anything else I played; I even thought I would pursue it as a career.

When I was 17 years of age, I weighed 275 pounds. Although I was only 5'11", the majority of my weight wasn't fat. I was much bigger than my peers, but I was fit and well-conditioned. Being large was an asset in football, where you need weight, strength, and speed to be successful—especially on the defensive line, where I played.

My senior year in high school was a turning point. I suffered a back injury that didn't stop me from playing, but it impeded my ability to train as I wanted. Even though I played injured my entire senior year, it was my best year ever. I was divisional MVP, defensive MVP, and all-state in Georgia for the 1995-1996 school year. My future seemed promising. I knew I was destined to play at the next level.

When the season ended, I needed to have surgery on my back. It was a routine surgery whereby a disc herniation would be addressed. I was told that I would be down for about 6 weeks, which would allow plenty of time to heal and prepare for spring training in college. I had many offers to play college football; my first choice was Duke University. It was always a dream of mine to play at the next level—the only thing standing in the way was my surgery.

I went into the hospital, and I was put under. That's when everything went wrong. To this day, no one fully understands what happened, but the doctor was forced to stop the surgery due to complications that couldn't be explained. He was unable to complete the procedure. When I entered the recovery room, I assumed all was well, but to my surprise, I was told the surgery wasn't successful. The first thing I wanted to know was, "When can I get the surgery again?" I assumed we could try it again soon—perhaps a week or two. Time was ticking and I needed to be 100% so I could report to camp. The doctor explained that he couldn't operate on me again until I healed 100%. I asked him how long would that take. He told me, "Six months."

I was crushed. It felt as if life had left my body. What would I do now? Life without football was a life I didn't want. Although it was devastating to me at the time, it was all a part of God's plan for my life. This point, at the end of my athletic career, is where my journey truly began.

When I stopped playing football, my appetite remained the same. I gained weight each year. At the height of my weight, I weighed 330 pounds. I got to the point that I hated what I saw in the mirror. I hated being overweight—having to shop for pants with a 46" waist meant that I had to go to specialty stores. I was always fearful of taking off my shirt at the pool or the beach. I always felt tired or in pain. Life was dismal. I was depressed, and I didn't like what I had become.

During my late 20s, I began to subconsciously identify with my condition. I accepted that being big was just who I was. Sometimes I would tell people, "It runs in my family." These were the things I did to keep myself in the place I had always been.

The mind plays tricks on us. When we see something we don't like, we start allowing ourselves to identify with it—to become wrapped up in our situation or circumstance. I never saw myself as a fit, healthy man, so I never allowed myself to think like one. The older I became, the more my health suffered. I developed more issues and problems. My knees were in pain, my back always ached, I was pre-diabetic, and I had high cholesterol. I went to the doctor and controlled my symptoms with pills and drugs. For many years, I thought this was my only option. So many others were on pills and prescription drugs, so I assumed this was the way. Every time I visited my doctor, there were never any other solutions offered to me. He never told me the importance of nutrition, or the many things I have come to learn. At the time, I thought my condition was normal.

The older I became, the worse my health was. I had to do something, but what that something was, I had no clue. One day, I woke up early in the morning and made up my mind that I would do something: I would start a new diet. Like most, I was excited: I set my date. When it came, I followed through. For days, I held fast to my diet, eating what I was instructed to eat and avoiding those things not a part of the plan. For a week, it worked; however, soon after, there I was, reverting to the person I had always been. I started eating all of the things I used to eat, and doing all the things I used to do. Not only did I gain back the few pounds I'd lost—I gained five more!

At this point, I gave up on change. I would just be who I was, I told myself. Being big was just part of being Joe. What else could I do, besides be content with that? Then, out of the blue, I received a phone call from eight-time Mr. Olympia Lee Haney. He said he had something to talk to me about. I was in my early thirties at this time, and a full-time pastor. Mr. Haney came to my office and met with me about his new program. The I.A.F.S. (International Association of Fitness Science) was a program designed to certify people in fitness science and nutrition. Mr. Haney told me he wanted me to join. He expressed the need for community, and how pastors are a major key to having this important conversation. I happily accepted the challenge, paid for the course, and trained with him.

Not only did I learn what to do while working out, but I learned the basics of nutrition. During my time with Mr. Haney, I learned what a protein, a carbohydrate, and a fat was. I learned what they did and how the interacted chemically within the body. I learned what happened if you mixed certain foods with other foods. My knowledge of nutrition broadened—I was a sponge, soaking up everything I could learn. Once I finished the program, I applied what I learned on myself. I changed what I ate—without telling anyone. Each day, I prepared my meals understanding what I was eating, and what it was doing to my body when I ate it. The moment I began to apply the knowledge I'd learned, weight started dropping quickly!

I had never lost weight like this. Each week, I was noticeably smaller. Many people close to me thought I was ill, or that something was wrong. When they asked me if I was okay, I told them that the weight loss was intentional. Each week, a new person would ask me what I was doing, and if I could help them, as well…I couldn't believe it!

In six months, I lost 60 pounds. I'd never felt so good! My energy levels increased, my power surged, and my blood work indicated to my doctor that I was healthy! I felt like superman! I was so excited because, to me, it felt like I had done the impossible. Before this, I had always felt unable to control what

I ate or when. Now I was calling the shots. I was casting my own destiny!

As time progressed, I continued to lose weight. Each month, I dropped more and more. Each month, I became more muscular and fit! Every Sunday after church, members would ask me to help them. I was becoming an authority on weight loss when, just eighteen months before, I had been 330 pounds! At this time, I knew I needed to take what I had learned and present it to others who needed it, but how could I execute something like this with masses of people? This was the challenge ahead of me.

Inception of the Journey: Divine Inspiration

When I knew it was my task to share my knowledge with others, I had no idea where to start. I didn't know of any other pastors who were in the space I was in; what I felt needed to be done did not exist. At the time, I felt that this was a problem, and I didn't know how to overcome it.

One day, while at a local coffeehouse, thoughts rushed into my mind. I quickly grabbed a napkin and began to write what was coming to me. On the napkin I wrote "Mind, Body, and Spirit." Of course, I was familiar with that concept; however, the inspiration I received was more dynamic. When I wrote those words on the napkin, I had a vision in my mind of what people needed and how it could be given to them.

Mind: Address how people think and what they focus on. Before anything else can be done, the power and ability of the mind must be taught. I needed to help people see that their focus creates their reality. Then, they could purge their lives through practices such as reflective blogging. The more negativity they unearthed, the more they would be primed for transformation!

I had never heard of the term "Reflective Blogging." I didn't know what it meant, nor did I read it from other sources. It was giving to me by God at that moment, and it was something I knew I needed to do. Instead of a person chronicling their actions during the day, I could teach them to blog reflectively. People need to understand not only what they feel, but why they feel it. "Happy" and "sad" are terms we use to describe how we feel; most people believe that there are external variables that result in happiness or sadness. I knew people needed to unearth the true "why" behind the "what."

Body: Every person needs to adjust their eating regimen in a way that maximizes energy and minimizes inflammation. The way I'd been eating during my transformation was the same way others needed to eat. I took my diet and structured it in a way that taught people *how* to eat, instead of telling them *what* to eat.

Every person I worked with would eat in the same philosophical way. I would teach them nutrition, and empower them to never be on a diet again. I was not selling a fad diet; I was empowering people to create a sustainable lifestyle.

Spirit: God should be the center of all things. This was, is, and will always be my belief. As people are transforming, God must be not only a part of that transformation, but the very essence of it.

Every day, each person I worked with would be focused on spiritual recalibration. Most of the people I worked with were Christians; however, my terminology was not religious.

I knew that what people needed was bigger than the church. Although Christ is the essence of who I am, I knew there are those who may view God in different ways. I never fought that and, at the same time, I never changed the essence of my beliefs. Even if there were people who were not Christians, I would happily work with them, and do my best to meet them where they were.

I looked at the napkin and realized I had my road map. I knew what I needed to do, and I knew that it was divinely inspired. Programs start and end; however, what God had given me was a process—something that never ends! Although I am a teacher, I still am learning, because the process of growth is ongoing.

Does the Process Work?

Once I'd developed the process, I knew I needed to test it. Would it work? How would people respond to it? At this point, I didn't know. In the summer of 2012, I assembled a group of 22 people. It was made up of 16 men and 6 women. All participants went through the 40-day "Mind, Body, and Spirit" process. I decided to name this process "The Journey."

For the first two days, all the participants would detox together. I created my own detox strategy that allowed people to flush their bodies of the harmful substances within. I always start with detoxing before I change a person's nutritional profile. This is most effective because it makes a new nutritional profile easier to adapt to, instead of eating a certain way one day and drastically changing someone's diet the next. With a two-day detox, the participant craves whatever new foods they eat. When the detox is over, they are happy, and they feel accomplished. This creates a powerful moment that pushes them through the days ahead.

I hired a professional statistician: Roland Wellmaker of the Morehouse School of Medicine. He took the participants and created measuring tools for each part of the process. Wellmaker assessed weight, cholesterol, waist circumferences, mental clarity and happiness, and spiritual connectivity to God. The tests were conducted before and after the process in order to properly assess the efficacy of The Journey. I had no clue what test results would be. When the 40 days had passed, the post tests were issued. Once Dr. Wellmaker processed the data, we saw in each category (physically, emotionally, and spiritually) that the process was statistically effective.

This gave me a great tool to share with others. Not only did the process pass the "eye" test, but it was now scientifically proven. I could move forward and maximize its results!

Holistic Medical Studies—Western Medicine

Now that I had established a working process, I wanted to do all I could to increase my knowledge so that I could educate and uplift those I served. My knowledge of nutrition was great, but I wanted more. I was attracted to holistic medicine; however, I didn't know what specific path to take.

All my life, I knew there was something fundamentally wrong with the practice of Western medicine. When we become sick or ill, we go to the doctor, tell him or her what hurts, and we're given a pill or prescription. There are so many people with preventable illnesses who are not empowered to heal themselves by altering their lifestyle. For years, this didn't make sense to me; but the older I became, the more I began to understand. The bottom line to Western medicine is this: the sicker people are, and the more medicine can be used to pro-long life, the more money the industry will make. This means more money for pharmaceutical companies, hospitals, insurance companies, treatment centers, and so on. I understood the medical industry from a business perspective, but why treat a person with Type 2 Diabetes with insulin when you can empower them to heal through lifestyle? The answer is simple: recovery presents a conflict of interest to the medical industry. If a diabetic heals himself of his condition, he no longer needs insulin or doctor visits.

One hundred million Americans are either diabetic or pre-diabetic.[8] When you think about that from a financial perspective, this means 1 in 3 Americans are paying for insulin, or will soon be paying for the treatment of a condition that can be eliminated (or controlled) through lifestyle changes. The medical industry has no incentive for people who are diabetic to not be diabetic. This philosophy can be applied to the treatment of almost any condition—even those deemed "incurable." Western medicine doesn't aim to heal patients, but rather to treat their conditions over an extended period of time for maximum profit. It's not incentivized to heal, but monetized to treat.

What attracted me to holistic medicine was its philosophic approach to health and wellness. Instead of treating a symptom, holistic medicine teaches us to avoid sickness by strengthening the body naturally. Good nutrition must be a part of this strategy. This is what I needed—because of that, I sought to complete my holistic studies.

---

[8] "More than 100 million Americans are living with diabetes or pre-diabetes." www.cdc.gov https://www.cdc.gov/media/releases/2017/p0718-diabetes-report.html. Accessed Jan. 8, 2020.

The Negative Stigma of Holistic Medicine

In the United States, medicine can only be practiced by doctors who have the proper credentials. This is an attempt to protect the public against those who aren't qualified, and it's a good protective measure. However, if you are a holistic or naturopathic doctor, you are oftentimes ostracized for several reasons.

First, holistic medicine is the practice of healing the person, not treating the symptom. This is the opposite of Western medicine's business model. If a holistic doctor is helping a person reverse diabetes, lower cholesterol naturally, or lose weight without gastric surgery, that doctor is taking money out of the circulation and control of Western medicine. This means that the more holistic doctors are ostracized, or considered "quacks," the better it is for business.

Second, natural remedies and vitamins cannot be patented. Any prescription drug that is designed and manufactured is patented by the pharmaceutical company, who will reap the benefits of the drug when it is sold and used. When doctors prescribe drugs to patients, many times it's because they're provided with "kickbacks" or incentives to promote that product.

No one owns a patent on vitamin C. Although there are proprietary mixtures and blends exclusive to certain companies, vitamins and minerals cannot be patented. For this reason, the back of the vitamin container will say, "The contents of this bottle have not be reviewed by the FDA."

Finally, when a doctor is able to help someone eat in a way that empowers them to avoid a future diagnosis, it greatly impacts the bottom line of pharmaceutical companies. For these reasons, holistic medicine is designed to prevent disease instead of treating the symptoms; and for that, it often gets a bad reputation in traditional medical circles.

Benefits of Being a Pastor in the Health and Wellness Space

When I began to work with people in the health and wellness space through The Journey, there were things about it I didn't like. I didn't want, for example, to be the "healthy" preacher. I did not want my peers to see me differently. For this reason, I never talked publicly about my work. I never shared the testimonials of people losing 40 pounds in 38 days, or the testimonies of people who were once diabetics and alcoholics who had healed themselves by changing their lifestyles. I never embraced what I was doing, and the lane God had me in.

As time progressed, the results continued. Every group who came through The Journey were the recipients of results that exceeded our highest expectations. The testimonials and support continued to pour in, group by group. Soon, I realized why it was so successful: the model created was based on results, not on profit!

People who participated in The Journey received better results than they had on other popular diets they'd paid for or subscribed to. We had some doctors who even sent patients to The Journey because of the results others received. People who suffered from alcoholism, drug addiction, and a litany of other psychological and emotional issues were able to address all of their problems through one process! It was at this point that I realized we had something the world needed. I fully embraced what we were doing, committing to do my best to help as many people as we possibly could.

Chapter 4
JUMPING INTO THE JOURNEY

In 2012, when The Journey first began, I had no clue what I was doing. I had never studied transformation from a clinical vantage point. I didn't know if the structure of the small groups (10-12 people each) was ideal. Nothing like it existed; for that reason, I started with what I had and learned as I went. As we progressed in the early sessions of The Journey, I learned a lot about people, their issues, and the things that inspire them. All of this knowledge has helped me understand this sphere of personal transformation. Here are just a few of the lessons I've gathered along the way.

Controlled Competition is Powerful

Human beings have an innate sense of competition. It's the reason for our love of sports all over the world. When Journey participants were placed into groups, one of the requirements to graduate was to lose 10 pounds. I require this because there needed to be some way of physically measuring a person's progress. Although weight is not always an indicator of health, within this context, it has its place.

As the process began, I noticed that people were focused on losing the weight. They wanted to do whatever they could to meet their goal; in many instances, this included not being outdone by their peers. Initially, I thought competition would pose a problem; however, as time progressed, I saw it become a great intrinsic motivational element that could be harnessed for good. If a person can allow competition to positively influence them to change their habits, it can actually help them!

Sometimes, competition backfired. After all, some people are intimidated by the success of others, especially when their own performance has not been optimal. Whenever this occurred, people would withdraw, or even drop out of the process. In certain situations, I was able to help these people see that their intimidation was not due to not the success of others, but their own lack of effort. When the participants tried harder to get results, their intimidation of others subsided. Of course, there were some situations in which this did not apply; however, overall I noticed competition becoming a positive tool that motivated people to change. Challenges and group competitions trigger an innate, visceral emotion in humans that can be used for good when the situation is controlled.

Group Support

Over the past years—almost a decade—that I've been conducting transformative processes, I've learned a lot. One of the most common comments of participants once the process ends is, "I have tried to change many times, but I never could." Their struggles vary, from those who've tried losing weight to those with personal addiction. One of the key factors to their success is the relationships they build inside of the experience. In the early stages of The Journey, I learned the importance of mutual support, and it's something I want to examine here, as well.

The Buddy System

There are three different forms of support that a participant receives. Every person who comes through the process is placed with a buddy. The buddy system is one of accountability. When we set goals in life, who is helping to make sure we're following through with what we say we'll do? Each week, when millions of people attend church, a gym, or anything wherein the goal is personal growth and improvement, we need to ask who those people are accountable to. Without accountability, the rate of success drops significantly.

Most failures in life can be attributed to not only personal missteps but to not having accountability. People in The Journey were less likely to fail, give up, or not advance because their buddy was present to check on them and make sure they stayed on track.

Initially, when we started to create groups, I would match each person with someone opposite from them in some way—gifts, talents, strengths, and weaknesses. I would take a person who was very outgoing and place them with someone a bit more introverted. I would take an older person and pair them with a younger person. I would take someone organized and detailed and place them with a person who was different. These weren't scientific pairings, but they were meant to keep people from being paired with their friends or people they knew. The more comfortable a person is with their buddy, the less likely they are to explore and create new bounds. Complacency breeds consistency. I wanted to make people as uncomfortable as possible; I believe that to be a major part of The Journey's success.

I noticed partnerships becoming powerful forces. The pairs were able to lean on one another's strengths while helping each other with their weaknesses. The old were able to give wisdom to the young, while the young were able to give energy and new perspective to the old.

The Group Itself

Human beings are tribal in nature. We enjoy groups, social environments, fraternities, sororities, and social clubs, just to name a few. Being a part of a group makes us feel safe and secure; this stems from a type of survival instinct—we move towards one another.

If a person desires to lose weight, they first make a decision that it's something they need to do. Second, they must decide the method for how they will lose the weight. Finally, they must follow through, or execute their plan of action. When the person starts, they are alone, figuring it out as they go. The endless times they are tempted with cheating make it harder and harder to stay faithful; however, when that same person is part of a group, they receive support and comfort they wouldn't have otherwise.

A participant in a group knows that everyone else is being tempted, just as they are. This can actually help them stay on track with their plan. As the group progresses together, there will be times when one person is weak, and someone else has strength. These roles may switch often, but this camaraderie is invaluable—when you're alone, you must be strong at all times. This is why it's best to go through the process of changing and developing one's willpower while in the safety of a small group.

As groups progress together, day by day and week by week, an energy is created that cannot be put into words. It's synergistic in nature. The progress of one person carries over to the next person. People feel like a part of the group, in some instances, more than they feel their own strength and resolve. The group becomes a control mechanism for the person who may not have those same positive relationships elsewhere. After all, not everyone who comes through the process has needed support from their spouse, friends, or work environment. The small group provides an environment of positivity and support, where people with like minds can serve as motivators to one another.

The Group Leader

Each group within the process has a leader. This person is the captain, responsible for keeping the group motivated and focused on the end goal. Each day, the group leader champions the efforts of the group in reaching their self-set goals; he or she gives the group what they need to be successful, whether that be emotional support or technical guidance.

At the beginning of the process, each group leader shares his or her testimony about coming through the process. This allows the participants to connect with them, as well as see someone who has done what they are trying to do. Along the way, this leader is able to fully identify with the struggles and obstacles of each participant. This is a powerful component to the success of the process. The more weeks that pass by, the more equity the leader has, as well. This means there is a level of influence others may not have; a special bond is created during the process, both from participant to leader and from leader to participant.

I remember one group that came about three years after The Journey's start (circa 2014). One of its participants started off strong and vibrant. This person was enthusiastic and excited about being in The Journey. For weeks, this participant was engaged, and displayed many characteristics of leadership. Near the end, however, the participant began to fade, and slowly withdrew from the group.

When the leader noticed this, they made contact with the participant, who shared that the issue was a domestic one. The leader happened to have a similar testimony, and gave the participant advice. The leader told them that their issues should not stop them from becoming a better version of themselves. This statement resonated strongly. The participant was able to make adjustments, and finished the process successfully. Today, that participant has been the leader of many groups, and has assisted in the transformation of many others.

As adults who have lives, jobs, careers, and responsibilities, we often neglect to seek out the support and attention we need. This small group model works because there are many levels of built-in support that assist someone in the transformation process.

Chapter 5

WHAT I LEARNED

After two years of six consecutive groups, around 2014, I began to learn a lot about transformative work—about people, their desire to change, and what they needed to change. These lessons have allowed me to formulate my own approach to transformative work, as well as to refine the process in order to help more people in the future. The things I learned are as follows.

Nutritional Cornerstone

Whenever I work with someone in transformation—in any capacity—I always begin by changing their diet. This is key to transformative work. If a person is looking to heal emotionally, spiritually, or physically, the food they're eating must be clean and nutritionally appropriate for what they are hoping to accomplish.

For example, if a person is suffering from alcoholism and desires to become sober (a difficult challenge, as we all can imagine), they will likely experience sugar cravings as they detox. These cravings are due to the absence of alcohol, which is quickly converted to sugar when ingested. The person will begin to crave sweets, like cookies, cake, and candy. This influx of sugar creates instability in the hormones, and leads to insulin spikes. When insulin is spiked, energy levels are affected, as well as a person's mood. If someone who desires to become sober is led through a process like The Journey, in which they are assisted with detoxing and given a new nutritional profile, it will take the edge off of these withdrawal symptoms.

When someone has fewer withdrawal symptoms, they are able to physically feel better. Their ability to sustain their sobriety increases exponentially. The bottom line is this: the better you feel, the easier it is to change mentally, physically and emotionally!

Break Down to Build Up

Something else I learned in the process of taking people through transformation is that must be a process of "breaking down," or being deconstructed, as well as a process of reconstruction. These words may appear harsh; however, when you look at the essence of transformation and what it is, that's exactly what happens.

When a person desires to change, they are essentially desiring to be someone different. Something has to stop, die, cease, or be removed for them to realize the transformation. If the process is attempted without understanding this, the changes will merely be temporary. Transformation *must* start with deconstruction.

If someone with an eating disorder goes on a diet—a program that tells them what and how to eat—they will see results over time. They will lose (or gain) weight, and will probably feel better about themselves; however, if the emotional and spiritual issues that drove them to eat (or to not eat) are not identified and dealt with, it's only a matter of time before the problem returns. All that has to happen is for the person to get off the diet—to have a "cheat" day or a relapse.

We must become aware of ourselves, how we feel, and what makes us do the things we do. Are we eating (or not eating) to feel better? To cope with issues? Out of habit? Awareness is the first step, because only at that point can it be controlled.

If a person who has an eating disorder discovers that they are moved to eat when they are stressed, this gives them a target to look for. Participants in The Journey are taught to notice what they feel *and* why they feel it. As this process is repeated, a person essentially destroys a part of themselves and reconstructs a "new" creature from within. This is the foundation of how I approach transformation. There must be a deconstruction and a reconstruction. If not, transformation cannot not truly manifest.

Needed Elements of Transformation

Since the inception of The Journey, I have been able to identify certain elements that people need to change. These elements are a part of every transformative process I've designed. Each element listed below is, in my opinion, intrinsic to personal transformation.

Direction

Every person, no matter their issues or obstacles, needs direction as to how to change. For a person who is obese, a clear diet or eating regimen is needed to take them where they need to be. There are many ways a person can lose weight; however, each individual needs a plan they can follow day by day. Likewise, a person who suffers from depression needs a plan of action to follow from point A to Z; they need guidance, structure, and a certain regimen to follow.

As you can see, this is essential to every transformative process, no matter what the issue is. Seeking change without a clear plan of action will not result in true transformation.

Support

When a person desires to change who they are in any way, support is essential in the process. Every person has some kind of support system, whether it be family, friends, or both. It's difficult to change when those closest to you aren't in your corner. If a person wants to give up smoking, but their friends are constantly asking them to smoke, their likelihood of success greatly diminishes.

In the past, there have been many who desired to adopt healthier lifestyles; however, those closest to them refused to transform with them. Because of the small group model, participants have the support they need that, to some degree, controls their environment. This model is essential and important to one's overall ability to change and receive the support they need.

Competition

Competition can be an excellent motivator within the process of transformation. As long as the competition is healthy, it can be used to inspire and evoke something within others needed to push them to a level they otherwise wouldn't reach.

By nature, people want what's best for themselves. This is a part of human nature that has allowed us to survive for millions of years. If my desire is to lose weight, improve my health, or develop myself as an individual, I want to accomplish that goal—that's my main motivation. Sometimes, during the process, a person loses their personal motivation. We've all been there: we stop eating properly, exercising, or doing whatever we need to do to make our goals manifest. This is when healthy competition kicks in and makes a difference.

Competition is external motivation. When I see others losing weight, progressing, or doing whatever I need to do, it can motivate me to change. I don't want them to change while I remain the same!

I've seen healthy coopetition move people beyond rough spots and hit benchmark goals. The only times competition becomes problematic is when it becomes someone's sole source of motivation. If the only reason you're is motivated to do something is to compete with someone else, then your desire to change isn't about what *you* want, but about that other person.

Momentum

One of the most common questions I've been asked during the last eight years is, "What motivated you to lose your weight and keep it off?" I never have to think long about my answer: "Results!"

When I started my process, I was more than 330 pounds. When I learned how to eat and what to eat—when I set my plan of action—I stuck to it every day. My commitment manifested amazing results in a short amount of time. I could see visible weight loss in my arms, legs, face, and waist. I felt better, lighter, happier, and stronger. One month in, I had lost 30 pounds—more than I'd ever lost at any given time before. I was thrilled and excited about my progress, and this caused my commitment and desire to grow. The more I lost, the more goals I surpassed.

When I weighed less than 300 pounds, I remember going to the mall one day and finally buying a regular pair of jeans. This was life changing for me! I was in the department store crying—people probably thought something was wrong with me; but everything was right! When I reflect on those milestones, I remember what I felt. I had gained momentum, and that's what kept me committed to my process. Each time I hit a goal, I wanted more. I wanted to see how far I could go!

Results create momentum. Momentum is what people need to keep them in the process. Why? Because they're able to see that the process works! They realize they are that much closer to their goals than they probably realized. I've witnessed thousands of people come through The Journey—people who said they could never lose weight dropped 40 pounds in 38 days. People who were on insulin for years came off of it. People addicted to drugs and alcohol freed themselves of the bondage of addiction in six weeks. In all of these cases, their personal victories were trophies used to keep them motivated. Not only were they motivated to finish their race, but they were motivated to never return to where they had been.

Setting Specific Goals

At the beginning of The Journey, I always ask each participant, "Why are you here?" This is a simple question, but a very important one. The goal is to help the person know exactly what they want out of the process.

Many will state tasks and objectives, not knowing what "success" truly looks like for them. When you start a project, you must know exactly what your target is. Why? So that you can constantly remain aware of where you are, how far you are from the goal, and what you need to do to get there in the time frame you've set for yourself. It's important to focus on a specific, clear goal—whether it's losing weight, living a healthier lifestyle, dealing with depression, or not being on prescription drugs, it's essential to set specific benchmarks by which you can measure your success.

When I started my journey, I wanted to lose 50 pounds. That was my ultimate goal at the time. Every week, I weighed myself. I was told by many professional and trainers not to do this. They said the scale doesn't always tell the right story. Although they have good points, the scale still tells an important story! For me, this was my way of tracking progress. I needed to see how far I'd progressed. I needed to know when I hadn't hit my goal, when I'd exceeded my goal, or even when I'd hit certain plateaus. When you set a goal and you don't hit it, it's not the end of the world; however, it does give you an indication as to the adjustments you need to make to get where you want to be.

Progress reporting is a major part of transformation. A person who desires to change needs to set their goal, and have ways to measure their progress. This is important not only for meeting goals but also for maintaining goals once they're met.

My Philosophy

As stated earlier, every transformative process in which I have assisted people started with my own journey. There were many things I did that were right, and there were many things I did that were wrong. My ultimate goal when I work with a person is to teach them how to relive their life. This can be difficult, but it is powerful when done correctly.

My philosophy of transformation is quite simple:

One: A person cannot change unless they are the **sole driver** of their own transformation. For this reason, I have never worked with a person who was brought to The Journey by someone else. They have to express their own personal desire to change. When that happens, their mindset is different, and they're able to focus. Without this focus, change is impossible.

Two: Transformation cannot be **compartmentalized**. This means that, if you desire to change your mind, you must make changes to your body, as well. If you desire to change your body, you must change your mind. Transformation must be holistic.

Three: Personal transformation is best done within the context of a **small group**. The group serves as a microcosm of a person's life: it has intrinsic needs, and every person within the group needs to change, as we've already discussed.

Four: **Education** is key. A person absolutely must learn about his or her issue, and how to fix it. My goal is to not only help get rid of the issue, but teach the person how to find, address, and remove it *for themselves*. When you allow education to be the foundation of the transformative process, each person's results become more sustainable.

PART 3
IT'S YOUR TURN

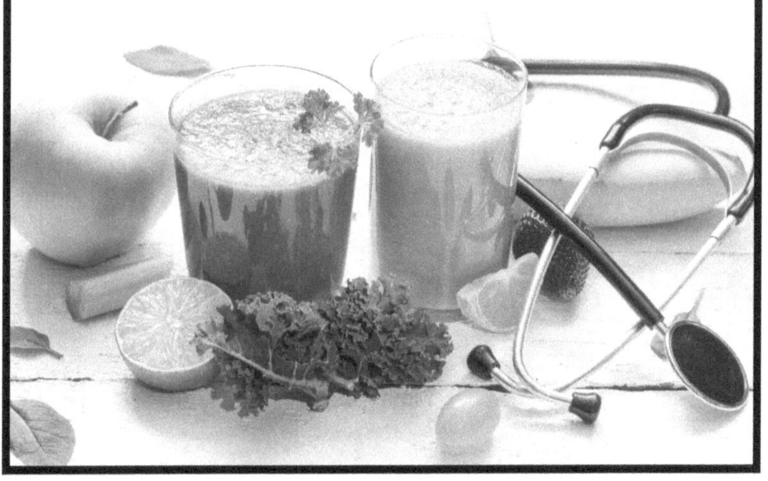

Chapter 6

THE 10 LAWS OF PERSONAL TRANSFORMATION

At this point, you hopefully find yourself in one of two groups: Maybe you've read about our forty-day transformative process, and you want to be a part of it; or maybe you're a person who's identified a needed area of change that you desire to tackle on your own. Regardless of where you are, the key is the desire to change. You have to move in a direction that will allow you to become the best possible version of yourself.

If you desire to change, it's important to reflect on "The 10 Laws of Transformation" I will share with you now. I have studied these laws, and deem them as necessary for a person to change, regardless of what the change is, or how challenging it's perceived to be. If you take these laws into consideration and apply them to your life, you will be well on your way to a brand new you!

1. Mastery of Mindset

Your mindset is the most important factor of your ability to change. It sets the effort you exert, your willingness to pursue your goal, and your desire to learn from your mistakes. For eight years, I never marketed The Journey to any person. Those who were in need always found me. I received emails from people across the country who needed help and wanted to change, but didn't know where to start. The issue with assisting a person isn't their lack of knowledge, but rather the mindset they are willing to adopt.

Some people show up desiring change, and they're in love with the outcome; however, they aren't willing to put in the work and sacrifice to realize their goals. A mindset for change is an important step that every person needs before any type of transformation can occur.

What exactly does it mean to have a "mindset for change?" It means you are willing to open your mind to things you haven't done, or things you may not see the value of in the beginning. I can remember seeing this firsthand in two different case studies.

The first time I saw it was with a middle-aged woman who had suffered from obesity all of her life. She had failed many times in her attempts to lose weight. When she contacted me, I placed her in a group; she didn't want to eat as I had instructed. She wanted to incorporate juices and smoothies into her diet, telling me about their health benefits and how her trainer thought it was good for her.

I knew the reasons for her obesity, but she did not. Drinking smoothies and other sweet juices, no matter how healthy they are, can be devastating for a person who is insulin resistant. Her body was in a constant state of fat storage, but she didn't understand that. For three weeks, she resisted my guidance, until one day, she decided to change her ways and follow my instructions perfectly. She lost 28 pounds in three weeks. Today she has lost more than 70 pounds.

The second time I saw this principle was with a man who had also been obese his entire life. He asked me to help him, and I even traveled to meet with him and give him his directives. He was excited about his change. Before beginning The Journey, he had a conversation with me and told me he wanted to do everything *except* be in a group; he wanted to do it on his own.

I told him the reasons for the small groups, but he still refused. His emotional issue was that he could not accept accountability. He was an accomplished man who had never been told "no." Sometimes, people like this allow their success to become their failure. He didn't want to help the group, and he didn't want to receive help. Everyone else in his group ended up losing massive amounts of weight, reversing their diabetes, and eliminating hypertension; however, he remained where he was.

These two case studies shared the same issue: their "mindset" was not focused on winning and being victorious. Before you start, you must be willing to focus on your goals, and never let anything cause you to waiver. When you desire change, the steps you have to take may not be consistent with what you think you should do. Trust the process. Keep going. Do what you need to do to change your life.

2. Clarify Your Goal

Whenever you begin a transformational process, you should never "just do it." It's better to start with a goal in mind. Ask yourself, "What am I trying to accomplish?" What this does is set a goal, as well as provide insight as to your progress toward it. If my desire is to become healthier, the question is, "How I will test my results? How will I know when my goal has been achieved?" Maybe I want to lose 20 pounds, lower my blood pressure by 20%, and reverse my diabetes within a period of three months. When goals are clearly set *before* the process begins, it allows you to focus on your objective and give it your all.

There was a time I set a goal to lose 30 pounds in 40 days. I started the process quickly, losing 10 pounds in the first week! I was excited about my progress, and assumed it would be just as easy for the remainder of the weeks. As time progressed, however, the weight dropped more and more slowly. Halfway through the process, I was more than 50 percent away from my goal. I reflected upon my goal, analyzed my plan of action, and tightened loose ends in my daily habits. I was *determined* to meet my goal. After I made these changes, I began to see noticeable shifts. The weight continued to fall, and I was able to reach my goal within my time frame!

The only reason I was able to reassess my progress was because I had a clear goal. This principle can be applied in the context of any goal you desire. The important thing is to set a clear goal. It doesn't even matter if you hit the goal or not; what's important is that you set a goal and do all that you can to achieve it.

When setting goals, it's also essential to set an obtainable goal—one that isn't too hard or too easy. If you set a goal that's unreasonable, or one you're not fully committed to pursuing, you're desiring something above your ability—this will lead to failure. Likewise, a goal that is too easy will breed complacency. A goal should be both attainable and difficult at the same time.

3. Accountability Partner

One of the hardest things in the world to do is change! To go against what you've done before—the patterns and habits you've created for yourself—can be quite difficult, to say the least. Most of the time, a person who desires to change will set a date to start; once it begins, they'll be successful in their efforts… until they aren't! How many times have you set a goal for yourself, only to get off the path at some point? Anything that keeps you from achieving your goal can be disastrous.

For this reason, we need partners who can progress with us through our process of transformation. This can be a spouse, friend, church group, or family member. When people are together and share a like mind and mutual focus, the strength of the group manifests as the strength of any person who needs it. When you become distracted or weak, your partner can motivate you to not give up. Sometimes, you may be the person who inspires your partner.

The mere fact I am in the space that I'm in keeps me accountable. How would those I influence feel if I let myself go? If I didn't live the life I preach about? Accountability has a powerful weight to it when used properly and intentionally.

When you select an accountability partner, you want to be sure it's the right person—someone able to do the following things:

Desire change for themselves. If you ask a person to be your partner or progress with you, no matter what that pursuit is, they must want to change for themselves—not for you! When it comes down to it, you aren't as important to them as they are to themselves. The person you select must want to change for themselves just as much as you want to change for yourself.

Be a good influence. You want a partner who is a good influence on you and your process. This doesn't mean they have to be perfect—just sincere in their efforts to attain their goals. Negativity can be draining, especially for person on a road to personal transformation. The start of the process will hold the greatest temptations. The better you are at starting strong, the more quickly you'll obtain good momentum that will lead you to your goal. Having a partner who is a good influence is key to the process.

Just as in any other relationship, a good accountability partner must be properly vetted. Take the time to not just pick a friend, but a partner—someone who will be invaluable to you as you strive towards your goal.

4. Don't Panic—Pivot

Four months after my personal journey, I had lost nearly 60 pounds. I felt better than ever, and knew I was out of the woods in terms of my struggles with obesity. I felt I had mastered my body: I knew what to eat, when to eat, and how to eat. I thought I had covered all of the bases I needed to be successful. For the first time since the start of my process, I was taking a much-needed vacation. Before, I had been home— everything I needed was right there. I was able to control my environment, which made it easier to stick to my daily habits.

For whatever the reason, I thought my trip would be just like home. When I arrived at my hotel, I was inundated with all types of welcome drinks, cookies, and deliciously-prepared foods that seemed so appealing. I felt just like the old me. I had no willpower, no control over myself. I was an emotional wreck, and I didn't know what to do. Instead of sitting down and thinking about all I knew to be true, I gave in to my temptations. I emotionally broke, and ate everything in sight! I gorged myself for days; when I returned home, I discovered I had gained 15 pounds in just a week's time.

Instead of pivoting and adjusting to my environment and situation, I panicked! I allowed my emotions to get the best of me. I folded and gave in to all my urges. I was so disappointed in myself, but I learned so much from this experience.

When you begin your process, your moment of panic will come. It will come at a moment when you least expect it. When it comes, embrace it, but see it for what it is: nothing more than the old you trying to retake its place in the driver's seat of your life. Instead of giving in, think and analyze your feelings. Pivot, and do whatever you need to do to make the right decisions. The next time I traveled, I learned from my mistake. I visited a local grocery store and filled my room with the foods I needed to make me feel comfortable and in control.

The point of this isn't what I did, but how I processed my feelings without allowing them to lead me in a direction I didn't want to go. When your time comes remember, don't panic—pivot!

5. Expect Resistance

When you make a decision to change yourself for the better, you would assume your choice would be respected and celebrated by everyone. You'd think that family members, friends, and those in your support circle will provide foundational encouragement. The sad reality is that this isn't always the case. People's actions and attitudes may not always be supportive. If you go into your journey not understanding this, it can derail your progress.

When I was 330 pounds, I felt loved and appreciated by many people. I had friends and folks around me whom I loved, and they loved me. When I made my decision to lose weight in order to enjoy a heather life, my relationships began to change—and it wasn't in the way that I would have expected. Whenever I'd go to social events, people who were my "friends" would get me to eat something they knew I shouldn't eat. They'd say, "This piece of cake won't hurt you," or, "Just eat a few wings—it won't make a difference." I couldn't understand why they would joke with me like this. When I would refuse to eat these foods, it would almost appear as if they were upset with me. I couldn't understand this for the longest time.

Now that I've seen this in the lives of those I've coached and assisted, I understand it. When people see you change and sacrifice the things you are to be who you desire to be, they often attempt to get you to deviate from your process. This is not always a conscious attack, but more so that others feel better about their own inability to change. In other words, when you eat the piece of cake, it makes them feel better about eating the cake they know *they* don't need. When you have the drink, it makes them feel better about the drink *they* are having.

When you refuse something they crave, love, or can't live without, your dedication reminds them of what they want to be but are not. This is a tough pill to swallow, but it's something you must understand. People like to connect with you in a way they remember, and they sometimes have no desire to connect with who you are trying to be. When I was overweight, I wasn't a threat to some of my friends; but when I

became fit, healthy, and bursting with confidence, it created envy in the lives of many whom I thought loved me.

The more you grow and the bigger your change, the more you will see this truth. When it comes, don't fear it—just understand it and see people for who they are. Remember, *any* person who is not 100% supportive of you being better, healthier, and happier isn't a person worthy to be your friend or a member of your support circle.

6. Start Fast, Start Strong

The transformative process requires energy and power. You are relearning how to live, how to think, and how to be. It's difficult to be something you haven't been! When a person decides to change, they must understand the gravity of the commitment. You have to put everything you have into the effort to change. The better you start, the higher your likelihood of success.

When a runner gets to the starting line, he prepares to run the race. He takes his mark, and prepares his mind and body for victory. The gun sounds, and he launches out of the gate. His form is perfect, his body is low to the ground as he progresses and generates his power, and he slowly begins to raise his view, all while sprinting towards the finish line. Many runners say the start is what determines how well you finish. The one who wins is the one who has the best start! As you prepare to change and transform, the same rule applies.

If you're not ready to give your transformation your all, don't do it! If you are not prepared to do everything you've set out to do, remain where you are! When you begin your process, you must be so focused and fixed on your goal that you won't let anything stop you from achieving it. In the first week of your process, like the runner, you will determine how you'll finish. It's so important that your focus is like a laser. This is the time to cross all your T's and dot all your I's. The first week isn't the time to slack or give it anything less than 100%. How you start is how you will finish.

When I went to college, I was told to work hard in order to have a good freshman year. Unfortunately, I didn't listen! I slacked, and didn't give my studies the time I should have. I finished my first year with a 2.5 GPA. I had to work for three years to raise my average. Had I started strong and fast, my sophomore, junior, and senior years would have been much easier, and I would have had more opportunities after I graduated.

The transformative process is the same. When you start, start strong and fast. Do all you can to nail your plan. Put all your energy and effort into it. Make up your mind that you won't stop until you get what you want.

7. Create and Sustain Momentum

The concept of the snowball effect is something many of us can picture: as a ball of snow begins to roll, it becomes larger and larger, and moves faster and faster. At a certain point, the snowball is moving so fast that it effortlessly grows and generates power because of its momentum.

We've already talked about the importance of forming and sustaining momentum, but it's worth mentioning again as part of the Top 10 Laws. Your process it will be difficult—everything you are trying to do is completely different than what you've done up to this point. You're exerting a lot of effort in the early days, because you are trying to start the process. The most important element of momentum is establishing it! This is why it's so important to follow your plan perfectly every step of the way. When you deviate from your plan, you hit "reset" on the momentum button.

If you are following a diet plan and you eat as you should for three days, then you cheat on the fourth day, you're saying to yourself, "Well it's no big deal. I'll just eat right next week." What you've done is actually negate what you did for the first three days of your diet. All the momentum you generated has stopped, and now you must start over!

There are three things you must keep in mind that will teach you how to create your momentum and how to sustain it. These are the last three laws of transformation.

8. Don't Cheat!

Whatever your plan of action is, stick to it. At all cost, don't deviate from it. If it's part of your plan, do it; if it's not part of your plan, don't do it. You don't realize how damaging it can be to you if you don't adhere to your plan.

All of the times I tried and failed to change were times in which I had no momentum. I'd start a diet for a day and cheat two or three days later. I would go to the gym for three days and then not go for a week. Cheating seems like it isn't a big deal, but trust me when I say that it is. You may not notice it right away; but at the end, it will all add up.

Let's say we have two cars, each of which are traveling 10 hours from one location to another. Car A leaves and makes one stop 5 hours into the trip. It takes Car A until 10:15 to arrive at his destination. Car B leaves at the same time, but each hour stops for gas, to stretch, or to take random pictures on the side of the road. Car B arrives at the same location 2 hours later than Car A. You can see how deviations add to the final destination time.

This works the same way when you're trying to transform; as you deviate from your plan, you leave results and progress on the table. When you start, don't cheat! Keep your focus and gain your momentum.

9. Enjoy the Ride!

When you start the process and you are able to continue for about two weeks (and not cheat), it will become easier and easier for you. Things that were difficult two weeks ago will now be easy. Things that were once a challenge will be second nature. The people who reach this state quickly are the ones who don't cheat!

When you feel the process of change getting easier and easier, it means you have good momentum. When this time comes, enjoy the ride. You will get your *best* results here! You will become healthier and feel energized because your consistency is carrying you in the direction you want to go. Get everything you can out of this stage, because it won't last forever!

10. Keep Your Foot on the Gas!

How many times have you seen a game on TV—whether it be baseball, basketball, hockey, or football—where one team had a huge lead, but as the game comes to an end, they end up actually losing the game? How does this happen? How can you lose such a big lead? It happens when you have momentum but you take your foot off the gas!

People who take their foot off the gas are people who play to lose, instead of playing to win. When you are ahead, and your results are manifesting, never be satisfied! Don't stop. Continue to be hungry, and desire to see more results. No matter how good you feel you're doing, keep your focus and continue to progress!

Chapter 7
ALWAYS LIVE IN REALITY

I remember the high I was in for those first months. I lost weight drastically; the pounds were falling off, because I had a plan that worked and I remained committed to it. Each day as I looked in the mirror and saw my results, I smiled, because I knew what it took to get them. I was committed to my journey, and I didn't just want to reach my goal, but to exceed it!

About four months into my process, I noticed my results began to slow down. I wasn't seeing the weight loss I once did. I didn't have the massive drops on the scale each week. I continued assuming it would change, or maybe it was just a "bad week." After about a month without seeing results, I became concerned. I didn't understand what was happening, and I didn't know what to do. All of my motivation was escaping me. I found myself in a plateau, and it was then that I began to say to myself, "Maybe this is where I need to stop." I began to question everything. Maybe the diet was wrong for me. Maybe I was just meant to be big!

I gave up. I didn't revert to my old self, but I remained at a state of no new results for several months. One day, I woke up, and it dawned on me why I'd hit a plateau! When I was 330 pounds, I set a goal for myself. I ate the same way and I exercised in the same way for 4 months. But now that I was fifty pounds lighter, if I wanted to lose more weight, I had to adjust the way I was eating and exercising.

I wasn't doing all I could. I had to be honest in order to move forward and get the results I wanted! I've watched people for years, in many processes of transformation, not be real with themselves. I've seen them give every excuse in the book—things that keep them from owning their own reality.

Those Who Question the Process

There are some people who question the process itself—whatever plan they use. I've seen people get results from a plan of action and hit a plateau; these people say things like, "This isn't for me." Remember, anything that got you results can continue getting you results. The problem isn't the process but whether we live in our own reality!

Those Who Question Their Own Limitations

There are some people who remain where they are because they feel that's all they can do. I've heard people say, "Being big is just who I am, because it runs in my family." Statements like this are not true. No matter what you read or what you hear, hypertension, diabetes, and obesity is not hereditary. What's hereditary are habits!

We must live in *reality*. The reality is, if you want something, you must be willing to work to get it! Questioning or doubting your ability is nothing more than an escape route for you to not try.

The Creation of Non-Negotiables

Results in life are always connected to the length of time certain habits are kept. This means that, if you want results in your transformation, you have to be consistent! This is the most important element of manifesting change. A person who has a subpar plan but is consistent will get better results than a person who has a stellar plan but isn't consistent.

When I started losing weight, there were many around me who told me I was losing weight too quickly. I've shared with you the reasons why they had this posture; however, this was something I didn't understand at the time. On one particular occasion, I remember a friend telling me I was obsessive, and that it wasn't healthy. She told me I would never take time off, even for my birthday or special holidays. She was right in that I never took breaks; however, she was wrong to tell me I was doing too much. I was creating a lifestyle that I felt was more important than my circumstances.

What is a non-negotiable, and how do we develop them? A non-negotiable is something you do no matter what—something you *never* compromise on. A good example is going to work. When you wake up, you never *really* ask yourself if you're going in. Maybe you don't want to go; but going to work (for most people) is a non-negotiable. When you get up on the morning on the days you are to be at work, you go! Another example is taking care of your children. When your kids wake up, they are in need of food and care. You never "take off" from caring for them, because you know that if you don't, no one else will.

Eating is a non-negotiable. We all need food to live and thrive. No matter what happens, you take time to eat. Perhaps you miss a meal here or there; but at the end of the day, you do it no matter what. Non-negotiables are the things you never consider not doing—you do them naturally.

The creation of non-negotiables is so important in the process of transformation. You must create things that you *never* deviate from. While on my transformative process, I created three non-negotiable that to this day I never deviate from!

My Nutritional Profile

When I am in a stage of maintenance as it relates to my weight, I will give myself two meals per week in which I eat whatever I want. Assuming I eat three meals per day, that's 21 meals per week, or 90% of my meals, that are completely planned. No matter what happens, I always adhere to this schedule.

If my birthday falls on a day when my "free meal" has not been allocated, I don't cheat! If special friends are in town and desire to go out, I will; however, I will not deviate from my diet. If 100 people ask me why I am not eating at a social function, it doesn't bother me. I don't get caught up on *anything* outside of my plan. The creation of a non-negotiable helps to keep me honest with myself, and makes it easier to never get into trouble.

My Workout Regimen

At this point of my life, I work out 6 days per week. Many people say this is too much; however, I love how exercising makes me feel. I am more accomplished, and I physically feel better when I work out. Each day is dedicated to a different routine. Three out of six days I spend on my bike, riding anywhere from 30-40 miles per session. On the other three days, I lift weights. No matter what, I always stick with my schedule.

The only thing that keeps me from riding outside is a lightning storm or inclement weather that could be harmful (like sub-freezing temperatures). When I travel, I pack the clothes

I need to work out in. If I'm on vacation, I work out. If it's Christmas Day, I work out. Holidays never keep me from my plan. This is a non-negotiable that I've kept, and will continue to keep, unless I am physically unable to fulfill it.

Weekly Fasting

Fasting is one of the most powerful practices a human being can do for their health, wellness, and mental clarity. Not eating does so much for the body in terms of healing and detoxification. The reason why you don't hear more people talking about fasting is because it's nothing to sell.

Since learning this principle and implementing it into my life, major changes have resulted. I've been doing this once per week. For a 24-hour period, I abstain from eating. All I consume is water during that time. There have been many things that have taken place on my fast day—holidays, birthdays, services, and travel. When it comes, I never deviate from my plan, because it is a non-negotiable I have created for myself.

You must create non-negotiables that extend past the time of your progress. If you only do them for six weeks or eight weeks, that's how long you will get results; but when you commit yourself to having non-negotiables as a part of your lifestyle, you will always have the life you want with the results you need!

Never Be Satisfied

When I started my process, I had a goal in mind. My desire was to wear size 38 jeans. For years, I wore a 44. At one point, I crept up to a 46. All I wanted was to be able to wear a size 38. That was my goal. I felt that, if I could reach it, I would never want anything else. If I were able to make that goal, I would have arrived.

It took me less than four months to go from a size 46 to a 38. When I reached my goal, I couldn't believe it. So many elements of my life changed. My self-esteem was through the roof. I felt better than I had in years. I'd accomplished something that had been a major obstacle for me.

After I reached my goal, I became a bit depressed. Perhaps you're reading this and you don't understand how I could go from being on top of the world to feeling down. I became depressed because I had reached the pinnacle (at least, what I felt was the pinnacle). I thought I had made it—there was nowhere else to go. When I looked at myself in the mirror, I was happy with my results; but I still wanted more. I wondered, "What if I could make it into 36 jeans?"

Finally, I decided that I wouldn't stay there—I would continue to move forward. Reinvigorated, I realized my journey wasn't coming to an end. I learned the power I was gaining: I had willpower to make myself do what I once was not able to do. I felt superhuman, and I didn't want this feeling to leave me. I went on to lose that extra seventy pounds. Although it took me more than a year, I continued to progress each and every month. People told me I was too small—that I didn't look healthy. People told me I needed to gain weight; but I didn't care what they thought or said. It wasn't their life—it was my life!

I reached size 34. I weighed 199 pounds. I couldn't believe what I had accomplished. Just think about what would've happened if I stopped when I hit my original goal. I would have left 70 pounds on the table; I would have left four additional inches on my waist. The point I'm making is, when you're able to reach your goal, *set another one*!

Today, I am almost 10 years into this space. I still challenge myself to do more and better than I have before. This is a spiritual thing that many people are not able to see. They think it's about the body, but it's actually about the mind and the spirit!

Today, I will challenge myself three times per year to accomplish something I have never done before. My weight was 199 pounds, but in 2019, I set a goal to hit my lowest weight ever. I got down to 196 pounds. This was huge for me, because it meant that I was hitting new milestones at the age of 42!

When you reach your goals, always apply this law: *Never* become satisfied! Always create goals for yourself so you can get better and better. Setting goals will do many things for you, including the following:

Goals Keep You from Reverting

I keep a photo in my phone that I look at whenever I can. In the photo, I was 330 pounds. When I started, I told myself I would never go back—I would never revert to the person I used to be. Many times, when we reach our goals, we will enter a mindset of rest and relaxation.

When we enter this state of mind, complacency creeps up on us, and we will find ourselves slowly releasing the reins. The old you will slowly creep back up; in many instances you can revert back to the person you never wanted to become again. When you keep goals in your life, it stops this reversion from occurring. Goals keep you going and growing in the right direction; they keep you engaged and motivated.

Goals Help You Become Your Best Self

When I lost my first 50 pounds or so, I thought I had arrived. When I made a conscious effort to continue, I lost an additional 70 pounds! The point is, when you continue to set goals for yourself, you continue to grow and evolve as a person.

I learned many things about myself that I wouldn't have known unless I continued. Losing the additional 70 pounds wasn't easy. I had to explore other eating plans and workout options. I dabbled in fasting, and studied insulin resistance and the hormonal impact of weight loss and weight gain. All of my knowledge was gained because I continued to set goals for myself.

The Spillover Effect

I've met many people who feel I am too serious, or an overachiever. Some people feel I'm always working, and will say various things about me that are complimentary to me but critiquing at the same time. Like I've said, this doesn't bother me, because I understand it. Continually setting goals for myself has changed me as a person. It's forced me to sacrifice comfort in my life. My outlook on work and dedication is different. Many times, when people find out what it takes to do something, they will veer away from it because it's difficult; however, I don't want to do anything unless it's hard!

This is a mindset I've been able to obtain in my personal journey. It applies to every element of life—even writing this book. It's the middle of the night right now, but I wanted to get this done. I wanted to finish it before the time I originally set for myself. It sounds crazy, but I've been able to do many things I wouldn't have done if I didn't have the capacity that I do. I'm no better than you, and I still have more to learn; but when you're continually setting goals, you are constantly growing.

CONCLUSION

I've shared with you the Ten Laws of Transformation. Each law is something I've seen at work within my own personal journey, as well as in the lives of thousands of others. If you apply these truths to your life and your transformative process, they will become a great asset for you.

You've heard my testimony and journey; you've been given information that, if applied, can transform you in any capacity you desire. Before we part, I want to share one final bit of information with you. I don't want to lessen the brightness of what I've shared with you, but I want you to understand this reality of life, and what you should expect during your transformative experience.

When I lost more than 130 pounds and established myself in the health and wellness space, I reached a place I never would have planned for myself. This often happens in God's plans for our lives. When I reached this space, many people looked up to me and took the words I told them as gold. For some, it was because I was their pastor; for others, it was because they saw my transformation for themselves. Nowadays, people have their eyes on me. People watch what I do and say. This places a lot of pressure on me; the people who feel that I have it all together don't understand what I go through behind closed doors!

You see, each day I wake up and take a journey that is a struggle. I have temptations each and every day. Sometimes, I wake up and I desire to eat things that aren't part of my plan.

Sometimes, I eat more than I should. Sometimes, all the willpower I have gained is lost, and I feel just as I did before! The old me is still there, deep down on the inside. My old desires and cravings have never completely left me. This is the truth of my story, and what you must understand: the old you will *never* die; it will always be there. I don't say this to discourage you, but to inspire you.

You may wonder, "If the old me is inside me, why should I think of transformation as a success?" Allow me to answer this question by sharing a story.

Several years ago, I purchased a dog for companionship as well as to help guard my home. The dog was a female Doberman pincher—I named her Storm. She was a fiery little thing, and I was so glad to have her. When I first got her, I spent time crate-training her, to be certain that accidents were kept to a minimum. As she got older, I noticed how rambunctious she was. She was always into things—biting my shoes, chasing the neighbor's cat, and getting into foods that weren't hers to eat! It got to the point that I called a professional trainer. The gentleman came to my home, assessed her, and told me what it would take to train her. He told me he would need six weeks with her, in a location different form my home. I wasn't expecting this at all; but once he explained the importance of the separation, I felt it made great sense.

For six weeks, I was without my new dog. I missed her and wanted her to return as quickly as possible. Finally, it was time for her to come home. I couldn't wait to have a brand new, fully-trained dog! I imaged what it would be like to have this perfectly behaved dog who listened to my command and did everything I asked of her. I couldn't wait to see her again.

The day arrived, and the trainer brought Storm back to my home. He placed a leash on her, and began to take her through a litany of training examples. She heeled, fetched, laid down, and rolled over—everything you could think of! It was an amazing presentation.

Once the session had ended, the trainer gave me his contact numbers and things to do if I had issues. When he left, I immediately took Storm to my friend's home to show them what she could do. I left the leash at home, because she had just been training for six weeks! When I got to my friend's home, many people from the neighborhood were all there. I just knew this was going to be a great presentation they would all be excited to see. I went through the tricks just as the trainer did with me; but to my surprise, Storm did none of them! I told her to sit, and she stood. I told her to come, and she ran away. I told her to heel. She acted as if I wasn't saying anything! I was livid; I had spent so much money, but all I had was a disobedient dog who was just as bad as she was before! I wanted my money back—I couldn't wait to call the trainer!

I called the trainer and asked him to come out that same day. I told him what happened, and he asked me to redo all the things that I did while over at my friend's house, so he could see the dog's behavior. I got the dog and did as he told me.

Before I could start, he asked me, "What are you doing? Where is the leash?"

I said, "It's in the house."

He began to shake his head. I had no clue what he was nodding at. He asked me, "Did you do all the commands with Storm without the leash?" I told him I had. He began to chuckle. "That's the problem, sir—you can't expect the dog to obey you without the leash. The dog was trained to obey commands with the leash on at all times. If you don't keep the dog on a leash, the dog will revert to who she was before being trained."

This is a story of transformation. Whatever you're seeking to change in your life, you are, in essence, retraining yourself to be something different. When you finish any process of transformation, the "old you" will always be there. It will never fully leave; for that reason, you must always keep the old you on a leash! If you don't, it will rise up and take over.

The way you keep the old you on a leash is by remembering these things:

Be consistent. Have a regimen in your life. Have a certain routine that you adhere to each and every day. No matter how much you desire to do other things or stray from your routine, keep it! The process of being regimented helps to keep the old you on a leash.

Objectively assess yourself at all times. If you desire to lose weight, weigh yourself to see if you're meeting your objectives. When you see the scale creeping upwards, it should be a signal that you need to get back in line and tighten up your daily routines.

Continue to set new goals. The more you make new goals for yourself, the more you'll suppress the old you. New goals cause you to direct your energy and focus in a way that keeps the old you in its proper place.

The secret of transformation is you that you will *never* become 100% what you desire to be. Anyone who tells you otherwise is not telling you the truth. If you're looking to become sober, you must *always* be aware of the old you. If you're looking for a healthier lifestyle, you must always be aware of the old you!

I've been doing this for ten years, and the old me still raises his head from time to time. The old me is still there, and will have a permanent address; however, I am the boss, and I now know that it's my duty to keep the old me on his leash!

Shalom.